# THE HERBALIST'S TOOLBOX: A COMPREHENSIVE GUIDE TO PRACTICAL HERBAL MEDICINE

*yoko coza*

ILLUSTRATED BY
THE AUTHOR

"The Herbalist's Toolbox: A Comprehensive Guide to Practical Herbal Medicine"

"The Herbalist's Toolbox: A Comprehensive Guide to Practical Herbal Medicine" is a comprehensive guide to herbal medicine that covers various aspects of herbalism. The book provides readers with practical advice on how to use herbs to treat a variety of health conditions, such as digestive issues, headaches, insomnia, and anxiety.

The book covers the different types of herbal preparations, such as infusions, decoctions, tinctures, and more, and provides detailed instructions on how to make these remedies at home. It also includes dosage and administration guidelines for different types of remedies and provides recommended herbs and dosages for various health conditions.

In addition, the book provides readers with essential tools and supplies for creating and administering herbal remedies. It covers the different methods of drying and preserving herbs, as well as tips for sourcing and purchasing high-quality herbs and supplies. The book also discusses the importance of sustainability and responsible harvesting when it comes to using herbs.

The book addresses the growing popularity of herbal

medicine in modern healthcare and emphasizes the importance of continued research and education in the field. Finally, it includes a list of resources for further learning and exploration in herbal medicine.

Overall, "The Herbalist's Toolbox" is an informative and practical guide for anyone interested in using herbs for their health and well-being. The book provides readers with the knowledge and tools they need to create and administer herbal remedies safely and effectively.

# chapter outline for "The Herbalist's Toolbox: A Comprehensive Guide to Practical Herbal Medicine"

1. Introduction to Herbal Medicine
- The history and philosophy of herbal medicine
- How herbal medicine works in the body
- The benefits and potential risks of using herbal remedies
2. Understanding Medicinal Plants and Herbs
- The types and parts of plants used in herbal medicine
- How to identify and classify medicinal plants
- The importance of sustainability and responsible harvesting
3. Growing and Harvesting Medicinal Plants
- Tips for growing and maintaining a medicinal herb garden
- How to harvest and store herbs for optimal potency
- The different methods of drying and preserving herbs
4. Preparation and Administration of Herbal Remedies
- The different types of herbal preparations (infusions, decoctions, tinctures, etc.)
- How to make herbal remedies at home
- Dosage and administration guidelines for different types of remedies
5. Herbal Remedies for Common Ailments
- A comprehensive guide to herbal remedies for various health conditions (e.g. headaches, digestive issues, insomnia, anxiety, etc.)
- Recommended herbs and dosages for each condition
- Possible side effects and interactions with other medications
6. Special Considerations in Herbal Medicine

- Herbal medicine for women's health issues (e.g. menstrual cramps, menopause, etc.)
- Herbal medicine for children and seniors
- The use of herbs in conjunction with other complementary therapies (e.g. acupuncture, massage, etc.)

7. Building Your Own Herbal Toolkit

- Essential tools and supplies for creating and administering herbal remedies
- How to create your own herbal first-aid kit
- Tips for sourcing and purchasing high-quality herbs and supplies

8. Conclusion: The Future of Herbal Medicine

- The growing popularity of herbal medicine in modern healthcare
- The importance of continued research and education in the field
- Resources for further learning and exploration in herbal medicine.

# CHAPTER 1:

## INTRODUCTION TO HERBAL MEDICINE

- ## *The history and philosophy of herbal medicine*

*Herbal medicine has been used by humans for thousands of years, and its history and philosophy are fascinating topics to explore. Here are three possible elements that could be included in a chapter on the history and philosophy of herbal medicine:*

1. *Origins of Herbal Medicine: The use of plants for medicinal purposes can be traced back to ancient civilizations such as Egypt, China, and India. Herbal medicine was also prevalent in traditional healing systems such as Ayurveda and Traditional Chinese Medicine (TCM).*

2. *Evolution of Herbal Medicine: Over time, herbal medicine has evolved and adapted to new cultures and changing medical practices. For example, during the Middle Ages, herbal medicine was practiced by monks who preserved the knowledge of medicinal plants, while in the Renaissance, herbalism became more scientific and experimental.*

1. Philosophies of Herbal Medicine: Many traditional healing systems, such as Ayurveda and TCM, view the body and mind as interconnected and seek to promote overall health and wellness. Herbal medicine is often used in conjunction with other modalities such as meditation, acupuncture, and dietary changes. The philosophy of herbal medicine emphasizes the importance of treating the root cause of illness rather than just managing symptoms, and seeks to support the body's natural healing processes.

- ### *How herbal medicine works in the body*

Understanding how herbal medicine works in the body is crucial for those interested in using or practicing herbal medicine. Here are three possible elements that could be included in a chapter on how herbal medicine works in the body:

1. Active Ingredients in Herbal Medicine: Many herbs contain active ingredients that have been shown to have specific effects on the body. For example, St. John's Wort contains hypericin, which has been shown to have antidepressant effects, while Echinacea contains echinacoside, which has been shown to boost the immune system.

2. Modes of Action: Different herbs work in different ways in the body. For example, some herbs may stimulate the production of certain hormones or enzymes, while others may have anti-inflammatory or antimicrobial effects. Understanding the modes of action of different herbs can help practitioners select the most appropriate herbs for a particular condition.

3. Interaction with the Body: Herbal medicine can interact with the body in a number of ways, including affecting the absorption and metabolism of other medications, stimulating or calming the nervous system, and supporting the liver's detoxification processes. Some herbs may also have a synergistic effect when combined with other herbs, leading to greater therapeutic benefit. Understanding how herbs interact with the body can help practitioners tailor treatment plans to individual patients and avoid potential herb-drug interactions.

- # *The benefits of using herbal remedies*

Herbal remedies have been used for centuries to promote health and wellbeing, and there are many potential benefits to using herbal medicine. Here are three possible elements that could be included in a chapter on the benefits of using herbal remedies:

1. Natural and Holistic: One of the main benefits of herbal medicine is that it is natural and holistic, meaning it seeks to support overall health and wellbeing rather than just treating symptoms. Many herbs have been used for centuries to promote health and prevent illness, and are believed to have fewer side effects than synthetic medications.

2. Personalized Treatment: Herbal medicine allows for a more personalized approach to treatment, as each herb has its own unique properties and effects on the body. Practitioners can tailor treatment plans to individual patients, taking into account their specific health concerns, lifestyle, and preferences.

3. Accessible and Affordable: Herbal medicine is often more accessible and affordable than conventional medical treatments. Many herbs can be grown at home or purchased at health food stores, making them an affordable and sustainable option for those who may not have access to traditional medical care. Additionally, many herbal remedies can be prepared at home, reducing the cost of treatment even further.

- ***potential risks of using herbal remedies***

While herbal remedies can offer many potential benefits, it's important to be aware of the potential risks and side effects associated with their use. Here are three possible elements that could be included in a chapter on the potential risks of using herbal remedies:

1. Herb-Drug Interactions: Herbal remedies can interact with prescription medications and over-the-counter drugs, which can lead to serious side effects or reduced effectiveness of the medication. For example, St. John's Wort, a popular herbal remedy for depression, can interact with many prescription medications, including antidepressants, birth control pills, and blood thinners.
2. Side Effects: Like all medications, herbal remedies can have side effects, especially when taken in large doses or over a long period of time. Some common side effects of herbal remedies include gastrointestinal upset, allergic reactions, and interactions with other medications.
3. Quality Control Issues: The quality and purity of herbal remedies can vary widely, which can affect their safety and effectiveness. Some herbal supplements may contain contaminants or adulterants, while others may not contain the advertised amount of active ingredients. It's important to purchase herbal remedies from reputable sources and to look for products that have been third-party tested for quality and purity.

# CHAPTER 2:

## UNDERSTANDING MEDICINAL PLANTS AND HERBS

- ### *The types and parts of plants used in herbal medicine*

Herbal remedies have been used for centuries to promote health and wellbeing, and there are many potential benefits to using herbal medicine. Here are three possible elements that could be included in a chapter on the benefits of using herbal remedies:

1. Natural and Holistic: One of the main benefits of herbal medicine is that it is natural and holistic, meaning it seeks to support overall health and wellbeing rather than just treating symptoms. Many herbs have been used for centuries to promote health and prevent illness, and are believed to have fewer side effects than synthetic medications.

2. Personalized Treatment: Herbal medicine allows for a more personalized approach to treatment, as each herb has its own unique properties and effects on the body. Practitioners can tailor treatment plans to individual patients, taking into account their specific health concerns, lifestyle, and preferences.

3. Accessible and Affordable: Herbal medicine is often more accessible and affordable than conventional medical treatments. Many herbs can be grown at home or purchased at health food stores, making them an affordable and sustainable option for those who may not have access to traditional medical care. Additionally, many herbal remedies can be prepared at home, reducing the cost of treatment even further.

- ## *How to identify and classify medicinal plants*

Identifying and classifying medicinal plants is an important skill for those interested in using or practicing herbal medicine. Here are three possible elements that could be included in a chapter on how to identify and classify medicinal plants:

1. Plant Anatomy: Understanding the anatomy of plants can be helpful in identifying and classifying medicinal plants. Some key plant parts to look for include the roots, stems, leaves, flowers, and fruits or seeds. Additionally, understanding the unique characteristics of different plant families can help in identifying specific medicinal plants.

2. Field Identification: There are a number of characteristics to look for when identifying medicinal plants in the field. These may include the size and shape of the plant, the color and texture of the leaves and stems, the presence of flowers or fruit, and the scent or taste of the plant. It's important to use a field guide or consult with an experienced practitioner to avoid misidentifying plants or mistaking toxic plants for medicinal ones.

- ### *The importance of sustainability and responsible harvesting*

Sustainability and responsible harvesting are crucial aspects of herbal medicine that are often overlooked. As demand for herbal remedies continues to grow, it's important to ensure that we are using these resources in a way that is environmentally sustainable and socially responsible.

One of the main reasons why sustainability and responsible harvesting are so important is that many medicinal plants are at risk of overharvesting or extinction. This is particularly true for plants that are in high demand, such as Ginseng and Goldenseal. Overharvesting can lead to a decline in the plant population, which can have serious ecological and economic consequences.

In addition to environmental concerns, there are also social and ethical considerations to take into account. Many of the communities that rely on medicinal plants for their livelihoods are also some of the most vulnerable and marginalized groups in society. Ensuring that these communities are able to benefit from the use and sale of medicinal plants is crucial for promoting social justice and economic sustainability.

There are a number of steps that can be taken to promote sustainability and responsible harvesting in herbal medicine. One important approach is to support organic and biodynamic farming practices, which prioritize soil health and biodiversity. Another approach is to source herbs from suppliers who prioritize sustainability and ethical sourcing practices, such as fair trade and regenerative agriculture.

Another important step is to promote education and awareness about the importance of sustainability and responsible harvesting. This includes educating consumers about the impact of their purchasing decisions, as well as supporting initiatives that promote sustainable and responsible harvesting practices.

Ultimately, promoting sustainability and responsible harvesting is not only important for the health of the planet and the well-being of marginalized communities, but also for the long-term viability of herbal medicine as a practice. By taking a proactive and responsible approach to herbal medicine, we can ensure that these resources will continue to be available for generations to come.

# CHAPTER 3:

## GROWING AND HARVESTING MEDICINAL PLANTS

- ***Tips for growing and maintaining a medicinal herb garden***

Growing and maintaining a medicinal herb garden can be a rewarding and enjoyable experience. Here are three possible tips for getting started and maintaining a successful herb garden:

1. Choose the Right Herbs: Before you start planting, it's important to choose the right herbs for your garden. Consider which herbs are best suited to your climate and soil type, as well as which herbs will be most useful for your needs. Some popular medicinal herbs to consider include Lavender, Chamomile, Echinacea, and Calendula.

2. Provide the Right Growing Conditions: Once you've chosen your herbs, it's important to provide the right growing conditions to ensure that they thrive. Most medicinal herbs prefer well-drained soil and plenty of sunlight, although there are some exceptions. Make sure to water your herbs regularly, especially during dry spells, and consider using organic fertilizers or compost to provide the nutrients they need.

3. Harvest and Store Your Herbs: Once your herbs are ready to be harvested, it's important to do so carefully and at the right time. Depending on the herb, this may involve harvesting the leaves, flowers, or roots. It's important to use clean, sharp tools to avoid damaging the plant, and to harvest during the right season for each herb. Once you've harvested your herbs, store them in a cool, dry place to preserve their potency and freshness.

Additional tips for maintaining a successful herb garden might include rotating your crops, companion planting to deter pests, and keeping an eye out for common plant diseases or pests. With the right care and attention, your medicinal herb garden can provide you with a bounty of natural remedies and healing plants for years to come.

And here are 30 tips for growing and maintaining a medicinal herb garden:

1. Choose herbs that are well-suited to your climate and soil type.
2. Plant your herbs in well-drained soil with plenty of organic matter.
3. Make sure your herbs get plenty of sunlight each day.
4. Water your herbs regularly, especially during dry spells.
5. Use organic fertilizers or compost to provide the nutrients your herbs need.
6. Mulch around your herbs to help conserve moisture and suppress weeds.
7. Prune your herbs regularly to encourage new growth and prevent disease.
8. Avoid over-watering, as this can lead to root rot and other problems.
9. Use natural pest control methods, such as companion planting and beneficial insects.
10. Rotate your crops each year to prevent soil-borne diseases.
11. Harvest your herbs at the right time for each plant, taking care not to damage the plant.

12. Dry your herbs thoroughly before storing to prevent mold and spoilage.
13. Store your herbs in a cool, dry place away from light and moisture.
14. Label your plants so you can easily identify them.
15. Keep a gardening journal to track your progress and successes.
16. Choose plants that are native to your area, as they are often better adapted to local conditions.
17. Experiment with different planting arrangements, such as raised beds or container gardening.
18. Take advantage of vertical space by planting climbing herbs or using trellises.
19. Use organic, non-toxic pest control methods to avoid harming beneficial insects and wildlife.
20. Choose disease-resistant varieties when possible.
21. Keep an eye out for common plant diseases and treat them promptly to prevent spread.
22. Test your soil regularly to ensure it has the right pH and nutrient levels.
23. Consider companion planting to deter pests and promote healthy growth.
24. Use natural mulches, such as straw or leaves, to conserve moisture and suppress weeds.
25. Consider incorporating herbs into your landscape design for both beauty and function.
26. Use compost tea or other natural fertilizers to boost plant growth and health.

27. Take time to observe your plants regularly to spot problems early.
28. Use crop rotation to prevent nutrient depletion and soil-borne diseases.
29. Consider growing herbs in a greenhouse or other protected environment for year-round growing.
30. Enjoy the process and don't be afraid to experiment and learn as you go!

- # *How to harvest and store herbs for optimal potency*

Harvesting and storing herbs properly is essential to preserving their potency and ensuring that they retain their medicinal properties. Here are some tips on how to harvest and store herbs for optimal potency:

1. Harvest at the right time: The best time to harvest herbs depends on the specific plant and the part of the plant that you are harvesting. In general, you want to harvest when the plant is at its peak potency. For example, you might harvest leaves before the plant flowers or seeds when the plant is in full bloom.

2. Choose the right tools: Use sharp, clean tools to harvest your herbs. Pruning shears, scissors, or a sharp knife are all good choices. Avoid using dull or rusty tools that could damage the plant or introduce bacteria.

3. Harvest in the morning: Harvesting in the morning, after the dew has dried but before the sun is too hot, is generally the best time. This is when the plant's essential oils and active compounds are at their highest concentration.

4. Avoid harvesting in wet conditions: If the plants are wet from rain or dew, wait until they dry before harvesting. Moisture can lead to mold and other problems during storage.

5. Cut properly: Cut stems just above a leaf node, leaving enough of the stem for the plant to continue growing. Avoid cutting too close to the ground, as this can damage the plant's roots.
6. Handle gently: Handle the herbs gently to avoid bruising or damaging the leaves, stems, or flowers. Bruised herbs will lose potency more quickly.
7. Clean your herbs: Before storing your herbs, make sure they are clean and free of debris. Rinse them gently under cool water and pat dry with a clean towel or paper towels.
8. Dry properly: To dry herbs, tie them into small bundles and hang them upside down in a well-ventilated area out of direct sunlight. Once they are completely dry, remove the leaves from the stems and store them in an airtight container.
9. Store properly: Store dried herbs in airtight containers, such as glass jars with tight-fitting lids. Keep them in a cool, dark place away from heat and moisture. Avoid storing them in the refrigerator or freezer, as the humidity can cause them to deteriorate.
10. Label your herbs: Be sure to label your herbs with the name and date of harvest. This will help you keep track of their potency and ensure that you are using fresh herbs when you need them.
11. Use within a year: Dried herbs will retain their potency for up to a year if stored properly. After that, their potency will begin to decline. Be sure to use your herbs within a year of harvest for optimal results.

12. Don't crush until ready to use: To preserve the potency of your herbs, avoid crushing or grinding them until you are ready to use them. This will help to preserve their essential oils and active compounds.

By following these tips, you can ensure that your herbs are harvested and stored properly for optimal potency. Whether you are using them for cooking, teas, or herbal remedies, fresh and potent herbs are essential for the best results

- ***The different methods of drying and preserving herbs***

Drying and preserving herbs is an important step in maintaining their freshness, flavor, and medicinal properties. Here are some different methods of drying and preserving herbs:

1. Air Drying: This is the most common and traditional method of drying herbs. Simply tie small bundles of herbs together and hang them upside down in a cool, dry, and well-ventilated place. Make sure the herbs are not exposed to direct sunlight, as this can cause them to lose flavor and color. Once the herbs are completely dry, remove the leaves from the stems and store them in an airtight container.
2. Oven Drying: This method involves placing the herbs on a baking sheet and drying them in the oven at a low temperature, usually around 180-200°F. Spread the herbs out in a single layer and check them frequently to make sure they don't burn. Once they are completely dry, remove the leaves from the stems and store them in an airtight container.
3. Dehydrator: A dehydrator is a convenient tool for drying herbs quickly and efficiently. Simply spread the herbs out on the dehydrator trays and follow the manufacturer's instructions for drying time and temperature. Once they are completely dry, remove the leaves from the stems and store them in an airtight container.

4. Microwave Drying: This method is faster than air-drying but requires careful attention to prevent the herbs from burning. Place a single layer of herbs on a paper towel and microwave them for 1-2 minutes at a time until they are dry and brittle. Check them frequently to make sure they don't overheat. Once they are completely dry, remove the leaves from the stems and store them in an airtight container.

5. Freezing: Freezing herbs is an excellent method of preserving their flavor and nutrients. Simply chop the herbs finely, place them in an ice cube tray, and fill with water. Freeze the cubes and store them in an airtight container in the freezer. Add the frozen cubes directly to soups, stews, and other recipes as needed.

6. Infused oils and vinegars: Infused oils and vinegars are a great way to preserve the flavor and medicinal properties of herbs. Simply fill a clean, dry jar with your favorite herbs, cover them with olive oil or vinegar, and let them infuse for several days or weeks. Strain out the herbs and store the infused oil or vinegar in a clean, airtight container.

7. Herbal butters: Herbal butters are a delicious way to preserve the flavor of herbs for use in cooking. Simply chop your favorite herbs finely, mix them with softened butter, and shape the mixture into a log. Wrap the log in plastic wrap and store it in the freezer until needed.

In conclusion, there are many different methods of drying and preserving herbs, each with its own advantages and disadvantages. Whether you prefer air-drying, oven-drying, freezing, or any other method, the key is to make sure the herbs are completely dry and stored in a cool, dry, and airtight container. With a little care and attention, you can enjoy the flavor and medicinal properties of fresh herbs all year round.

# CHAPTER 4:

## PREPARATION AND ADMINISTRATION OF HERBAL REMEDIES

- ***The different types of herbal preparations (infusions, decoctions, tinctures, etc.)***

Herbs can be used in a variety of different ways to create herbal preparations, each with their own unique benefits and uses. Here are some of the most common types of herbal preparations:

1. Infusions: Infusions are made by steeping herbs in hot water, much like making a cup of tea. Infusions are typically made with delicate herbs, flowers, and leaves that are not boiled or simmered. They are a gentle way to extract the volatile oils and other beneficial compounds from the herbs. Infusions can be consumed as a tea, used as a facial steam, or added to bathwater.

2. Decoctions: Decoctions are similar to infusions but are made by simmering tougher plant parts such as roots, bark, and seeds in water for a longer period of time. Decoctions are typically made with herbs that have a woody or fibrous texture and require a longer brewing time to release their active compounds. Decoctions can be consumed as a tea, used as a mouthwash, or applied topically to the skin.

3. Tinctures: Tinctures are liquid extracts made by steeping herbs in alcohol or glycerin. The alcohol acts as a solvent, extracting the active compounds from the herbs and preserving them for long-term storage.

Tinctures are a potent and convenient way to use herbs, as they can be easily added to water, juice, or other beverages. Tinctures are also useful for herbs that are not easily soluble in water.

4. Capsules: Capsules are a convenient way to take herbs in a standardized and controlled dosage. Herbs are ground into a fine powder and encapsulated in a gelatin or vegetarian capsule. Capsules are particularly useful for bitter herbs or herbs with a strong taste that may be difficult to consume in other forms.

5. Salves and ointments: Salves and ointments are topical preparations made by combining herbs with a base of beeswax and oil. The herbs are infused into the oil, which is then melted with beeswax to create a semi-solid consistency. Salves and ointments can be used to treat skin conditions, bruises, and other topical ailments.

6. Poultices: Poultices are topical preparations made by grinding fresh or dried herbs and applying them directly to the skin. Poultices are typically used to treat bruises, sprains, and other acute injuries. They can be made by wrapping the herbs in a piece of cloth or gauze and applying them directly to the affected area.

7. Essential oils: Essential oils are highly concentrated extracts made by distilling herbs with steam or water. They are highly potent and should be used with caution, as they can cause skin irritation if not properly diluted. Essential oils can be used in aromatherapy, massage, and other topical applications.

In conclusion, there are many different types of herbal preparations, each with their own unique benefits and uses. Whether you prefer infusions, decoctions, tinctures, or any other method, the key is to choose the right preparation for the herb and the desired effect. With a little experimentation, you can find the perfect herbal preparation for your needs.

# • *How to make herbal remedies at home*

Making herbal remedies at home is a rewarding and cost-effective way to take control of your health and well-being. Here are some steps to follow when making herbal remedies at home:

1. Choose your herbs: The first step in making herbal remedies is to choose the herbs you want to use. Be sure to do your research and select herbs that are safe and appropriate for your needs.

2. Gather your materials: Depending on the type of herbal remedy you want to make, you will need different materials. For example, if you want to make a tea, you will need dried herbs, hot water, and a strainer. If you want to make a tincture, you will need herbs, alcohol, and a glass jar.

3. Prepare your herbs: Once you have your herbs and materials, it's time to prepare your herbs. If you are making a tea or infusion, you will need to steep the herbs in hot water for a certain amount of time. If you are making a tincture, you will need to chop the herbs and soak them in alcohol for several weeks.

4. Strain and store: After your herbal remedy has steeped or infused for the appropriate amount of time, it's time to strain and store it. Use a strainer or cheesecloth to remove the plant material from your tea or infusion. If you are making a tincture, strain the liquid through a fine mesh strainer or coffee filter. Store your herbal remedy in a dark, cool place, away from sunlight and heat.

Here are some common types of herbal remedies you can make at home:

1. Herbal teas and infusions: Herbal teas and infusions are a simple and effective way to consume herbs. To make a tea or infusion, steep the herbs in hot water for 5-10 minutes, then strain and drink.

2. Tinctures: Tinctures are made by soaking herbs in alcohol for several weeks, then straining and bottling the liquid. Tinctures are a potent way to consume herbs and can be added to water or taken directly by mouth.

3. Salves and balms: Salves and balms are topical herbal remedies made by combining herbs with a base of oil and beeswax. The herbs are infused into the oil, then melted with beeswax to create a solid consistency. Salves and balms can be applied directly to the skin to soothe and heal.

4. Herbal syrups: Herbal syrups are a sweet and tasty way to consume herbs. To make an herbal syrup, simmer the herbs in water until the liquid is reduced, then add honey or sugar to taste. The syrup can be consumed by spoonful or added to water or other beverages.

By following these simple steps, you can easily make your own herbal remedies at home. With a little experimentation and creativity, you can find the perfect herbal remedies for your needs and preferences.

- ### ***Dosage and administration guidelines for different types of remedies***

When it comes to taking herbal remedies, it is important to follow dosage and administration guidelines to ensure safety and effectiveness. Here are some general guidelines for different types of herbal remedies:

1. Herbal teas and infusions: Herbal teas and infusions are generally safe and gentle, but it is still important to follow dosage guidelines. A typical dose is one cup of tea or infusion, consumed up to three times a day. Steep the herbs in hot water for 5-10 minutes, then strain and drink. For more potent remedies, you can increase the amount of herbs or steep them for a longer period of time.

2. Tinctures: Tinctures are a potent way to consume herbs and should be taken in smaller doses. A typical dose is 30-60 drops of tincture, taken up to three times a day. Tinctures can be added to water or taken directly by mouth. Always dilute tinctures for children and those with sensitive systems.

3. Capsules and tablets: Capsules and tablets are convenient and easy to use, but it is important to follow dosage guidelines. Read the label carefully and follow the recommended dosage. In general, a typical dose is one or two capsules or tablets, taken up to three times a day.

4. Salves and balms: Salves and balms are topical herbal remedies and should be applied directly to the skin. Follow the instructions on the label for application guidelines. In general, apply a small amount of salve or balm to the affected area and rub in gently.

5. Herbal syrups: Herbal syrups are a sweet and tasty way to consume herbs. Follow the instructions on the label for dosage guidelines. In general, a typical dose is one or two teaspoons of syrup, taken up to three times a day. Syrups can be consumed by spoonful or added to water or other beverages.

It is important to note that everyone's body is different, and dosage guidelines may need to be adjusted based on individual needs and sensitivities. Always start with a lower dose and gradually increase as needed. If you experience any adverse effects, stop using the herbal remedy and consult with a healthcare provider.

In summary, following dosage and administration guidelines is essential for safe and effective use of herbal remedies. Be sure to read the label carefully, start with a lower dose, and adjust as needed. If you have any questions or concerns, consult with a healthcare provider or a qualified herbalist.

# CHAPTER 5 :

## HERBAL REMEDIES FOR COMMON AILMENTS

- ***A comprehensive guide to herbal remedies for various health conditions (e.g. headaches, digestive issues, insomnia, anxiety, etc.)***

Herbal remedies have been used for centuries to treat a variety of health conditions. Here is a comprehensive guide to some common health issues and the herbs that can help alleviate symptoms:

1. Headaches: Headaches can be caused by a variety of factors, including stress, tension, dehydration, and allergies. Herbs that may help alleviate headaches include feverfew, peppermint, lavender, and ginger.

2. Digestive issues: Digestive issues such as bloating, gas, and constipation can be uncomfortable and disruptive. Herbs that may help alleviate these symptoms include ginger, fennel, peppermint, chamomile, and dandelion root.

3. Insomnia: Difficulty falling or staying asleep can have a negative impact on overall health and well-being. Herbs that may help promote relaxation and sleep include valerian root, passionflower, chamomile, and lavender.

4. Anxiety: Anxiety can manifest in a variety of ways, from general unease to panic attacks. Herbs that may help alleviate anxiety symptoms include ashwagandha, lemon balm, chamomile, and lavender.

5. Colds and flu: Colds and flu can be uncomfortable and disruptive to daily life. Herbs that may help alleviate symptoms include echinacea, elderberry, ginger, and garlic.

6. Menstrual cramps: Menstrual cramps can be painful and disruptive to daily life. Herbs that may help alleviate menstrual cramps include ginger, turmeric, chamomile, and black cohosh.

7. Joint pain: Joint pain can be caused by a variety of factors, including inflammation and arthritis. Herbs that may help alleviate joint pain include turmeric, ginger, devil's claw, and willow bark.

8. Respiratory issues: Respiratory issues such as coughs and congestion can be uncomfortable and disruptive. Herbs that may help alleviate respiratory symptoms include thyme, licorice root, eucalyptus, and marshmallow root.

It is important to note that while herbal remedies can be effective for some people, they are not a substitute for medical advice and treatment. It is always best to consult with a healthcare provider before starting any new herbal remedies, especially if you have any underlying health conditions or are taking medications. A qualified herbalist can also provide guidance on the appropriate herbs and dosages for your individual needs.

## • ***Recommended herbs and dosages for each condition***

Please note that herbal remedies should always be used with caution and under the guidance of a qualified healthcare provider or herbalist. The following are some common herbs and dosages that have been used traditionally for various health conditions:

1. Headaches:
- Feverfew: 50-150mg of a standardized extract daily
- Peppermint: 1-2 teaspoons of dried leaves steeped in hot water, 3 times per day
- Lavender: 1-2 teaspoons of dried flowers steeped in hot water, 2-3 times per day
- Ginger: 250mg of a standardized extract, 2-4 times per day

2. Digestive issues:
- Ginger: 1-2 teaspoons of fresh grated ginger root steeped in hot water, 2-3 times per day
- Fennel: 1-2 teaspoons of crushed seeds steeped in hot water, 2-3 times per day
- Peppermint: 1-2 teaspoons of dried leaves steeped in hot water, 3 times per day
- Chamomile: 1-2 teaspoons of dried flowers steeped in hot water, 2-3 times per day
- Dandelion root: 1-2 teaspoons of dried root steeped in hot water, 2-3 times per day

3. Insomnia:
- Valerian root: 300-600mg of a standardized extract, taken 30-60 minutes before bedtime
- Passionflower: 0.5-2 teaspoons of dried herb steeped in hot water, 2-3 times per day
- Chamomile: 1-2 teaspoons of dried flowers steeped in hot water, 2-3 times per day
- Lavender: 1-2 teaspoons of dried flowers steeped in hot water, 2-3 times per day

4. Anxiety:
- Ashwagandha: 300-500mg of a standardized extract, taken 2-3 times per day
- Lemon balm: 1-2 teaspoons of dried herb steeped in hot water, 2-3 times per day
- Chamomile: 1-2 teaspoons of dried flowers steeped in hot water, 2-3 times per day
- Lavender: 1-2 teaspoons of dried flowers steeped in hot water, 2-3 times per day

5. Colds and flu:
- Echinacea: 300-500mg of a standardized extract, taken 2-3 times per day
- Elderberry: 1-2 teaspoons of dried berries steeped in hot water, 2-3 times per day
- Ginger: 1-2 teaspoons of fresh grated ginger root steeped in hot water, 2-3 times per day
- Garlic: 1-2 cloves, minced or chopped and mixed with food or taken as a supplement

6. Menstrual cramps:
- Ginger: 1-2 teaspoons of fresh grated ginger root steeped in hot water, 2-3 times per day
- Turmeric: 400-600mg of a standardized extract, taken 2-3 times per day

- Chamomile: 1-2 teaspoons of dried flowers steeped in hot water, 2-3 times per day
- Black cohosh: 20-80mg of a standardized extract, taken once per day

7. Joint pain:

- Turmeric: 400-600mg of a standardized extract, taken 2-3 times per day
- Ginger: 1-2 teaspoons of fresh grated ginger root steeped in hot water, 2-3 times per day
- Devil's claw: 500

- ***Possible side effects and interactions with other medications***

While herbal remedies can be beneficial for many health conditions, it's important to be aware of potential side effects and interactions with other medications. Here are some examples:

1. St. John's Wort: Often used as a natural treatment for depression, St. John's Wort can interact with a variety of medications, including antidepressants, birth control pills, and blood thinners. It can also cause photosensitivity, making your skin more sensitive to the sun.
2. Echinacea: This herb is commonly used to boost the immune system and treat colds and flu. However, it can interact with medications that suppress the immune system, such as those used for organ transplants.
3. Ginkgo biloba: Known for its ability to improve memory and cognitive function, Ginkgo biloba can interact with blood thinners and increase the risk of bleeding. It can also cause gastrointestinal upset and headaches.
4. Valerian root: This herb is often used to treat insomnia and anxiety. However, it can interact with sedatives and other medications that cause drowsiness, making you feel more tired than usual.

5. Licorice root: Often used to soothe sore throats and calm coughs, licorice root can interact with medications that lower potassium levels, such as diuretics. It can also cause high blood pressure and edema if taken in large doses for extended periods of time.

It's important to speak with your healthcare provider before taking any herbal remedies, especially if you are taking prescription medications or have a chronic health condition. They can help you determine the appropriate dosage and potential interactions with your current medications. Additionally, be sure to purchase herbal remedies from reputable sources and follow package instructions carefully.

# CHAPTER 6 :

## SPECIAL CONSIDERATIONS IN HERBAL MEDICINE

- ***Herbal medicine for women's health issues (e.g. menstrual cramps, menopause, etc.)***

Herbal medicine has been used for centuries to address various women's health issues such as menstrual cramps, menopause, and hormonal imbalances. Many herbs contain properties that can help regulate and balance the female reproductive system, alleviate symptoms, and promote overall well-being. In this section, "The Herbalist's Toolbox: A Comprehensive Guide to Practical Herbal Medicine" provides an in-depth discussion of the best herbs for women's health and how to use them effectively.

The book covers common menstrual issues such as painful cramps, heavy bleeding, and irregular cycles. It provides a list of herbs such as cramp bark, red raspberry leaf, and ginger that can alleviate menstrual pain, promote hormonal balance, and regulate the menstrual cycle. The book also discusses herbal remedies for menopause symptoms such as hot flashes, night sweats, and mood swings. Herbs such as black cohosh, dong quai, and vitex have been traditionally used to reduce these symptoms, and the book outlines dosage and administration guidelines for each herb.

The section on women's health also covers herbs for fertility and pregnancy. It discusses herbs such as red clover, nettle leaf, and raspberry leaf, which are believed to improve fertility and prepare the uterus for pregnancy. The book also provides a guide to safe herbal use during pregnancy and how to address common pregnancy-related issues such as nausea, fatigue, and stress.

In addition to discussing the specific herbs for women's health, the book also covers the importance of holistic self-care practices such as stress management, exercise, and a healthy diet in promoting overall well-being. It emphasizes the importance of approaching women's health issues from a holistic perspective, considering not just the physical symptoms but also the emotional and mental aspects.

Overall, "The Herbalist's Toolbox: A Comprehensive Guide to Practical Herbal Medicine" provides a thorough and practical resource for women seeking natural remedies for their health issues. It emphasizes the importance of taking a holistic approach to women's health and provides a comprehensive guide to the best herbs and self-care practices to promote overall well-being.

- ### *Herbal medicine for children and seniors*

Herbal medicine can be a safe and effective way to promote health and wellness in both children and seniors. However, it's important to use caution when administering herbs to these populations, as their bodies may react differently to certain remedies.

Herbal Medicine for Children:

1. Chamomile: Chamomile is a gentle herb that can help calm fussy babies and toddlers. It can also promote restful sleep and relieve digestive discomfort.
2. Elderberry: Elderberry is a powerful immune booster that can help prevent colds and flu in children. It can also help reduce the severity and duration of symptoms if your child does get sick.
3. Calendula: Calendula is a soothing herb that can be applied topically to help heal minor skin irritations, such as diaper rash and eczema.
4. Ginger: Ginger can help relieve nausea and vomiting in children, especially those undergoing chemotherapy or experiencing motion sickness.
5. Echinacea: Echinacea can help boost your child's immune system and prevent or reduce the severity of colds and flu.

Herbal Medicine for Seniors:

1. Turmeric: Turmeric is a powerful anti-inflammatory herb that can help reduce pain and stiffness associated with arthritis.
2. Milk thistle: Milk thistle is a liver-supportive herb that can help protect against liver damage and improve liver function in seniors.

3. Hawthorn: Hawthorn is a cardiovascular-supportive herb that can help improve circulation and reduce blood pressure in seniors with heart conditions.
4. Ashwagandha: Ashwagandha is an adaptogenic herb that can help reduce stress and promote overall well-being in seniors.
5. Ginkgo biloba: Ginkgo biloba can help improve memory and cognitive function in seniors, making it a popular herb for those with dementia or Alzheimer's disease.

It's important to consult with a healthcare provider before administering any herbal remedies to children or seniors, especially if they have underlying health conditions or are taking prescription medications. Additionally, always follow package instructions carefully and purchase herbal remedies from reputable sources to ensure safety and efficacy.

- ***The use of herbs in conjunction with other complementary therapies (e.g. acupuncture, massage, etc.)***

Herbal medicine is often used in conjunction with other complementary therapies, such as acupuncture, massage, and chiropractic care. These therapies can work together to promote overall health and wellness, and may even enhance the effects of herbal remedies.

Acupuncture and Herbal Medicine: Acupuncture is a traditional Chinese medicine practice that involves the insertion of thin needles into specific points on the body. Acupuncture can be used to treat a variety of conditions, including pain, anxiety, and infertility. When used in conjunction with herbal medicine, acupuncture can enhance the effects of herbs and improve treatment outcomes. For example, acupuncture can help improve circulation and enhance the absorption of herbal remedies, making them more effective.

Massage and Herbal Medicine: Massage therapy is a hands-on therapy that involves the manipulation of muscles and soft tissues to promote relaxation and relieve pain. When used in conjunction with herbal medicine, massage therapy can help enhance the effects of herbs and promote overall well-being. For example, a massage therapist may use an herbal-infused oil or lotion during a massage to help promote relaxation and relieve muscle tension.

Chiropractic Care and Herbal Medicine: Chiropractic care is a healthcare practice that focuses on the musculoskeletal system, particularly the spine. Chiropractic care can be used to treat a variety of conditions, including back pain, headaches, and sciatica. When used in conjunction with herbal medicine, chiropractic care can help improve treatment outcomes and promote overall health and wellness. For example, a chiropractor may recommend certain herbs to help reduce inflammation and promote healing after an adjustment.

Herbal medicine can also be used in conjunction with other complementary therapies, such as aromatherapy, yoga, and meditation. Aromatherapy involves the use of essential oils to promote relaxation and relieve stress. When used in conjunction with herbal medicine, aromatherapy can enhance the effects of herbs and promote overall well-being. Yoga and meditation can also be used in conjunction with herbal medicine to help promote relaxation, reduce stress, and improve overall health and wellness.

When using herbal medicine in conjunction with other complementary therapies, it's important to work with a healthcare provider who is knowledgeable about the use of herbs and their potential interactions with other therapies. Additionally, always follow package instructions carefully and purchase herbal remedies from reputable sources to ensure safety and efficacy.

In summary, the use of herbs in conjunction with other complementary therapies can help promote overall health and wellness and enhance the effects of herbal remedies. Whether you're using acupuncture, massage, chiropractic care, or other therapies, always work with a healthcare provider who is knowledgeable about the use of herbs and can help guide you in the safe and effective use of herbal medicine.

# CHAPTER 7 :

# BUILDING YOUR OWN HERBAL TOOLKIT

- ***Essential tools and supplies for creating and administering herbal remedies***

Creating and administering herbal remedies requires a variety of tools and supplies to ensure safety, efficacy, and consistency. Whether you're making herbal teas, tinctures, salves, or capsules, here are some essential tools and supplies you'll need to get started:

1. Mortar and Pestle: A mortar and pestle is a traditional tool used for grinding herbs into powder or breaking them down for infusions and decoctions. It's an essential tool for making herbal remedies from scratch and ensuring that the herbs are properly prepared for use.
2. Herb Grinder: An herb grinder is a convenient tool for grinding herbs quickly and efficiently. It's especially useful for grinding larger quantities of herbs for tinctures and capsules.
3. Strainer: A strainer is used to separate the herbal material from the liquid in infusions and decoctions. It's important to use a strainer with a fine mesh to ensure that all of the herbal material is removed from the liquid.
4. Cheesecloth: Cheesecloth is a versatile tool used for filtering and straining herbal material. It's especially useful for making tinctures and oil infusions, as it allows the liquid to pass through while retaining the herbal material.

5. Double Boiler: A double boiler is used for heating herbs and oils without overheating or burning them. It's essential for making salves, balms, and other herbal preparations that require gentle heating.

6. Glass Jars and Bottles: Glass jars and bottles are essential for storing herbal remedies, especially tinctures and oil infusions. It's important to use dark glass bottles to protect the herbs from light and ensure that the remedy remains potent and effective.

7. Labels: Labels are an essential tool for keeping track of your herbal remedies and ensuring that they are properly identified. Make sure to label each remedy with the name of the herb, the date it was made, and the intended use.

8. Measuring Spoons and Cups: Measuring spoons and cups are used to ensure accurate measurements when making herbal remedies. It's important to follow recipe instructions carefully to ensure safety and efficacy.

9. Funnel: A funnel is a useful tool for pouring liquid remedies into bottles and jars without spilling or wasting any of the precious herbal material.

10. Storage Containers: Storage containers are essential for storing dried herbs, especially if you grow your own herbs. Make sure to use airtight containers to protect the herbs from moisture and insects.

11. Capsule Filler: A capsule filler is a useful tool for making your own herbal capsules. It allows you to fill capsules with the precise amount of herbal material, making it easy to administer a consistent dosage.

12. Dropper Bottles: Dropper bottles are essential for administering liquid herbal remedies, such as tinctures and oil infusions. They allow you to measure and administer precise dosages, making it easy to adjust the dosage as needed.
13. Digital Scale: A digital scale is an essential tool for accurately measuring the weight of dried herbs and other ingredients. It's important to use a scale to ensure that the correct amount of herbs is used in each remedy.
14. Gloves: Gloves are an essential tool for handling herbs and other ingredients. They help protect your hands from irritation and ensure that the herbs remain clean and free from contaminants.
15. Blender: A blender is useful for creating herbal powders and smoothie blends. It allows you to mix herbs and other ingredients quickly and efficiently, making it easy to create delicious and nutritious herbal remedies.

When creating and administering herbal remedies, it's important to use high-quality tools and supplies to ensure safety, efficacy, and consistency. Whether you're a beginner or an experienced herbalist, investing in these essential tools and supplies will make the process of creating and administering

- ## *How to create your own herbal first-aid kit*

Creating your own herbal first-aid kit can be a great way to have natural remedies on hand for minor injuries and illnesses. Here are some tips on how to create your own herbal first-aid kit:

1. Choose a container: The first step in creating your own herbal first-aid kit is to choose a container that is durable and easy to carry. A small, sturdy box or bag with compartments can work well.
2. Stock up on basic supplies: Some basic supplies you should have in your herbal first-aid kit include bandages, gauze, scissors, tweezers, and a thermometer.
3. Choose herbs for common ailments: Depending on your specific needs, you may want to include herbs for common ailments such as cuts, scrapes, bruises, burns, and insect bites. Some herbs that are commonly used for these purposes include calendula, comfrey, plantain, lavender, and chamomile.
4. Include essential oils: Essential oils can be a great addition to your herbal first-aid kit. Tea tree oil is a popular choice for its antiseptic properties, while peppermint oil can help with headaches and nausea.
5. Don't forget about pain relief: For pain relief, you may want to include herbs such as arnica, St. John's wort, and willow bark. These herbs can help with pain and inflammation associated with minor injuries.

6. Consider your environment: Depending on where you live and the activities you participate in, you may want to include specific herbs in your kit. For example, if you live in an area with a lot of poison ivy, you may want to include jewelweed, which is known to be effective in treating poison ivy.

7. Be prepared for travel: If you plan to take your herbal first-aid kit with you on the go, make sure to include items such as hand sanitizer, sunscreen, and insect repellent.

8. Label everything: Make sure to label all of the items in your herbal first-aid kit, including the herbs and essential oils. This will ensure that you can easily identify everything and use it properly.

9. Keep it up to date: It's important to periodically check your herbal first-aid kit to make sure everything is still in good condition and hasn't expired. Replace any items that have expired or that you have used up.

Overall, creating your own herbal first-aid kit can be a great way to have natural remedies on hand for minor injuries and illnesses. With the right supplies and a little bit of preparation, you can create a kit that meets your specific needs and is easy to use in any situation.

- ***Tips for sourcing and purchasing high-quality herbs and supplies***

While herbal remedies can be beneficial for many health conditions, it's important to be aware of potential side effects and interactions with other medications. Here are some examples:

1. St. John's Wort: Often used as a natural treatment for depression, St. John's Wort can interact with a variety of medications, including antidepressants, birth control pills, and blood thinners. It can also cause photosensitivity, making your skin more sensitive to the sun.
2. Echinacea: This herb is commonly used to boost the immune system and treat colds and flu. However, it can interact with medications that suppress the immune system, such as those used for organ transplants.
3. Ginkgo biloba: Known for its ability to improve memory and cognitive function, Ginkgo biloba can interact with blood thinners and increase the risk of bleeding. It can also cause gastrointestinal upset and headaches.
4. Valerian root: This herb is often used to treat insomnia and anxiety. However, it can interact with sedatives and other medications that cause drowsiness, making you feel more tired than usual.

- ### ***Tips for sourcing and purchasing high-quality herbs and supplies***

1. Research reputable suppliers and read reviews from previous customers.
2. Look for suppliers that offer organic and sustainably sourced herbs.
3. Choose suppliers that follow Good Manufacturing Practices (GMP) for quality control.
4. Check the expiration date and freshness of the herbs before purchasing.
5. Consider purchasing whole herbs instead of pre-packaged blends to ensure purity.
6. Buy herbs in small quantities to ensure freshness and potency.
7. Purchase herbs in their proper form, such as fresh, dried, or powdered, depending on the recipe.
8. Avoid purchasing herbs from unknown sources, as they may be contaminated or mislabeled.
9. Choose suppliers that provide clear and accurate labeling, including the Latin names of the herbs.
10. Look for suppliers that offer a wide variety of herbs and herbal preparations.
11. Check for any certifications, such as USDA Organic, Non-GMO Project Verified, or Fair Trade Certified.
12. Consider purchasing herbs from local farmers or community-supported agriculture (CSA) programs.
13. Check the origin of the herbs to ensure they are not imported from countries with lax regulations.

14. Purchase herbs that are free from pesticides, herbicides, and other harmful chemicals.
15. Consider the cost of the herbs, but do not sacrifice quality for a lower price.
16. Look for suppliers that provide detailed information on the benefits and uses of each herb.
17. Ask for recommendations from trusted herbalists or health professionals.
18. Consider purchasing bulk herbs and supplies to save money in the long run.
19. Check for any potential allergens or interactions with other medications before purchasing.
20. Look for suppliers that offer educational resources, such as books or online courses.
21. Consider purchasing from suppliers that have a commitment to sustainability and reducing their carbon footprint.
22. Choose suppliers that offer a money-back guarantee or return policy.
23. Check for any additional fees, such as shipping or handling charges.
24. Purchase herbs and supplies from suppliers that provide excellent customer service.
25. Look for suppliers that have a positive reputation in the herbal community.
26. Check for any special certifications, such as Kosher or Halal.
27. Consider purchasing from suppliers that offer discounts for frequent buyers or bulk purchases.

28. Look for suppliers that have transparent sourcing and production practices.
29. Consider purchasing herbs and supplies from local health food stores or co-ops.
30. Choose suppliers that have a commitment to ethical and fair trade practices.

# CHAPTER 8:

## CONCLUSION: THE FUTURE OF HERBAL MEDICINE

- ### *The growing popularity of herbal medicine in modern healthcare*

Herbal medicine has been used for thousands of years in various cultures around the world, and its popularity has continued to grow in modern healthcare. With a focus on natural remedies and holistic approaches to healing, many people are turning to herbal medicine as a complementary or alternative therapy to conventional medicine.

One reason for the growing popularity of herbal medicine is the increased availability of information and education on the subject. The internet has made it easier for people to research and learn about different herbs and their uses, and there are now numerous online resources, books, and courses dedicated to herbal medicine.

Another factor contributing to the popularity of herbal medicine is the growing concern over the side effects and long-term health risks associated with some prescription medications. Many people are seeking natural alternatives that can treat their health conditions without the potentially harmful effects of pharmaceutical drugs.

In addition, the rise of integrative and functional medicine has also contributed to the popularity of herbal medicine. Integrative medicine combines conventional and complementary therapies to provide a more holistic approach to healthcare, while functional medicine focuses on identifying and treating the root causes of health issues rather than just addressing symptoms.

Furthermore, the increasing recognition and acceptance of herbal medicine by healthcare professionals and institutions has also helped to boost its popularity. Many healthcare providers are now incorporating herbal remedies into their treatment plans, and some hospitals and clinics offer integrative medicine programs that include herbal medicine.

The growing popularity of herbal medicine has also led to an increase in scientific research on the efficacy and safety of herbal remedies. While there is still much to be learned about the effects of herbal medicine on the body, numerous studies have shown promising results for the use of herbs in treating various health conditions, such as anxiety, depression, and chronic pain.

However, it is important to note that herbal medicine should not be used as a replacement for conventional medical treatments when necessary. While herbal remedies can be effective in treating certain health conditions, there are some cases where conventional medicine is necessary for proper treatment and management.

Overall, the growing popularity of herbal medicine in modern healthcare reflects a shift towards a more holistic and natural approach to healing. As more people seek alternative therapies and natural remedies, the role of herbal medicine in healthcare is likely to continue to grow and evolve in the coming years.

- ### *The importance of continued research and education in the field*

As the popularity of herbal medicine continues to grow, the importance of continued research and education in the field cannot be overstated. While herbs have been used for centuries for their medicinal properties, there is still much to be learned about their effects on the body, optimal dosages, and potential interactions with other medications. One of the main reasons why research and education are important is to ensure the safety and efficacy of herbal remedies. While many herbs are generally considered safe, some can have side effects or interact with other medications, making it important to have a thorough understanding of their effects on the body. By conducting research and providing education on the use of herbs, healthcare providers can help to ensure that patients are using herbal remedies safely and effectively.

In addition, continued research can help to identify new uses for herbs and improve our understanding of how they work in the body. For example, recent studies have shown promising results for the use of herbs in the treatment of conditions such as anxiety, depression, and chronic pain. By conducting further research, we can better understand the mechanisms by which herbs work and identify new applications for their use in healthcare.

Furthermore, education on the use of herbs is important to ensure that healthcare providers are able to incorporate herbal remedies into their treatment plans in a safe and effective manner. Many healthcare providers may not have a comprehensive understanding of herbal medicine, and may not be able to provide accurate guidance to patients who are interested in using herbs as a complementary therapy. By providing education on the use of herbs, healthcare providers can better serve their patients and provide a more holistic approach to healthcare.

Finally, research and education can help to combat the misinformation and myths that surround herbal medicine. There are many myths and misconceptions about the use of herbs, and it is important to provide accurate and evidence-based information to the public to help them make informed decisions about their health.

In conclusion, the importance of continued research and education in the field of herbal medicine cannot be overstated. By conducting research and providing education, we can ensure the safety and efficacy of herbal remedies, identify new uses for herbs, and provide accurate guidance to healthcare providers and patients. As the popularity of herbal medicine continues to grow, it is important that we continue to invest in research and education to help us better understand the potential benefits and risks of these natural remedies.

- ***Resources for further learning and exploration in herbal medicine.***

If you are interested in further learning and exploration in herbal medicine, there are many resources available to you. Here are a few suggestions:

1. Books: There are countless books on herbal medicine available, ranging from beginner guides to more advanced texts. Some popular titles include "The Herbal Medicine-Maker's Handbook" by James Green, "The Complete Medicinal Herbal" by Penelope Ody, and "The Modern Herbal Dispensatory" by Thomas Easley and Steven Horne.
2. Online Courses: Many online courses are available for those who want to deepen their knowledge of herbal medicine. Some popular options include the Herbal Academy, the American Herbalists Guild, and the School of Traditional Western Herbalism.
3. Conferences and Workshops: Attending conferences and workshops is a great way to learn from experienced herbalists and connect with other like-minded individuals. Some popular conferences include the International Herb Symposium and the United Plant Savers Medicinal Plant Conservation Conference.
4. Herbalists: Seek out local herbalists in your area and ask if they offer consultations or apprenticeships. Learning from a practicing herbalist can be an invaluable experience and provide a more personalized approach to learning.

5. Herbal Gardens and Farms: Visiting herbal gardens and farms can provide hands-on experience with different herbs and their growing habits. Look for botanical gardens or herb farms in your area and take a tour or attend a workshop.

6. Online Resources: There are many online resources available for those interested in herbal medicine, including blogs, podcasts, and websites. Some popular options include the Herbal Academy blog, the HerbRally podcast, and the American Herbalists Guild website.

7. Social Media: Many herbalists and organizations share information and resources on social media platforms such as Instagram and Facebook. Follow herbalists and organizations that align with your interests and values to stay up-to-date on the latest information and resources.

Remember to approach learning about herbal medicine with an open mind and a willingness to learn from a variety of sources. There is a wealth of knowledge and experience available in the world of herbal medicine, and with dedication and curiosity, you can deepen your understanding and appreciation of this ancient practice.